# HERPES

## A NUTRITIONAL APPROACH

by Louise Tenney, M.H.

© 1996

Woodland Publishing Inc.
P.O. Box 160
Pleasant Grove, UT 84062

The information contained in this book is in no way to be considered as prescription for any ailment. The prescription of any medication should be made by a duly licensed physician.

# TABLE OF CONTENTS

| | |
|---|---|
| HERPES: WHAT IS IT? | 3 |
| WHY VIRUSES ARE SO HARD TO KILL | 3 |
| TYPES OF HERPES | 4 |
| WHAT CAUSES HERPES | 5 |
| HOW DOES HERPES SPREAD? | 6 |
| HOW DOES HERPES DEVELOP? | 6 |
| WHAT FACTORS CONTRIBUTE TO THE DEVELOPMENT OF HERPES? | 7 |
| MENUS AND RECIPES | 25 |
| RECIPES | 27 |

# HERPES: WHAT IS IT?

If you are an individual who has been diagnosed with herpes, be assured that you are not alone. It is estimated that there are over 50 million herpes sufferers, and that rate is projected to increase at 500,000 new cases yearly.

Herpes can refer to any of a variety of conditions which usually result in the eruption of a blister. Forms of the herpes virus are responsible for miserable and annoying conditions, including cold sores which affect the lips and genital sores. Herpes is a virus therefore it is difficult to kill. Viruses are some of the most resilient microorganisms found in nature.

The bad news is that once herpes enters the body, it remains there indefinitely. Certain conditions seem to bring it out of dormancy, resulting in the formation of painful fluid-filled blisters. These blisters are considered highly infectious until they heal over, which usually takes three weeks.

In the case of genital herpes, sores can develop from two to seven days after contact and a recurrence of the blisters is common. The herpes virus seems to weaken after the age of fifty, when outbreaks become much less common.

# WHY VIRUSES ARE SO HARD TO KILL

Herpes is a virus and, unfortunately, once it gets into your system it stubbornly persists. The Herpes virus has plagued mankind for millennia. Viruses are very tricky and adaptive organisms. They are extremely small and can only be detected through powerful electron microscopes.

Technically, viruses can be considered parasitic. They cannot survive on their own and depend on a host organism for their survival. To avoid detection by the body's immune system, which would attempt to destroy it, the virus encases itself in a protein shell. Markers on the exterior of the shell, which would usually alert immune defenders-which would learn to recognize their codes-change frequently, confusing immune functions. Viruses subsequently enter a host cell, then sheds its protein coat. The virus integrates its DNA with the host cell's genetic code. The cell does nothing to extricate the virus, believing it is part of itself.

Once genetic reprogramming is set in motion, the cell's genetic system replicates viruses at a dramatic rate. This replication ultimately leads to the demise of the host cell due to its eventual bursting. These new viruses subsequently have the opportunity to spread throughout the body, invading more cells by repeating the cycle.

Although herpes viruses destroy some body cells, curiously, they can live in harmony with others. Scientists do not completely understand this phenomenon. They have described the herpes virus as being one of the most complicated viruses of our modern era.

# TYPES OF HERPES

**(1). HERPES SIMPLEX 1:** This variety of the herpes virus causes cold sores and fever blisters. If it spreads to the mucosa of the eye, it can cause serious damage, possibly resulting in ulceration of the cornea and subsequent blindness. Herpes Simplex can also cause encephalitis if it finds its way to the brain. Herpes Simplex 1 particularly likes to reside in the mucous membranes of the mouth area, and because of its affinity for these areas, it is known as the herpes virus which strikes above the waist.

**(2). HERPES SIMPLEX 2:** This form of herpes is also called "genital herpes" and has been referred to as the most common venereal disease in America. Genital herpes strikes below the waist. Women who have had this type of Herpes stand an increased chance of developing cancer of the cervix and vulva. Some clinical studies reveal that half of women with cervical cancer had previously been infected with herpes, which continues to invade the cancerous cells as well. The August, 1981 edition of the *New England Journal of Medicine* reported a connection between the escalating rate of cancer in female sex organs and the rising increase in the number of herpes infections. Women can be unaware they have genital herpes. This type of herpes can pose a significant threat to an unborn baby during pregnancy. Neonatal herpes has a high fatality rate.

(3). **VARICOLLAZOSTER:** This form of herpes causes chicken pox in children and can resurface later in life as shingles.

## WHAT CAUSES HERPES

The annoying blisters of herpes can break out when the immune system becomes compromised, which can occur during periods of intense stress. Stress factors can vary, from environmental exposure to sun or wind which causes chafing to wearing tight clothing or lack of sleep. Emotional stressors such as anger, grief and depression can also precipitate the eruption of herpes sores.

Immunosuppressive drugs can alter the body's defense system and trigger severe herpes infections which can, in some cases become fatal. Physiological contributors to herpes outbreaks include certain body temperature and blood conditions. Acid-producing foods seem to activate the virus while ingesting alkaline-promoting foods appears to keep the virus in a dormant state. Chinese medical practitioners believe that when the blood becomes too acidic, the human body become more susceptible to the herpes virus. For this reason, acid-forming foods should be eliminated. Some of these include: pineapple, citrus fruits, cherries, tomatoes and coffee. Arginine-rich foods should also be avoided. Apparently the herpes virus needs arginine, which is an amino acid, to conduct its metabolic processes. These foods include: peanuts, cashews, chocolate, cola, peas, cereals and beer.

# HOW DOES HERPES SPREAD?

The following are ways in which the Herpes virus can be spread:

- Herpes Simplex 1 can be contracted by kissing a contaminated person or eating off the same utensil etc. (any time a saliva exchange can occur).

- Herpes Simplex 2 is usually transmitted via sexual contact.

# HOW DOES HERPES DEVELOP?

The pattern for herpes development consists of stages:

**(1).** The first stage, which is contagious, is announced by a numbing, itching or tingling sensation in the affected area during a period of 12 days. Sometimes an overall tired, sick feeling is also present.

**(2).** The second stage, which is also contagious, is manifested by the appearance of clusters of greyish, fluid filled blisters.

**(3).** The third stage is non-contagious and occurs when the blisters scab over.

## WAYS TO DECREASE THE SPREAD OF HERPES

Dr. Jill E. Ferguson, M.D., and Halvor L. Harley, III., M.A., J.D., in their book *Herpes Sufferers Get H.E.L.P,* outline steps to prevent the spread of herpes:

- 1. Recognition is vital in stage 1. Learn to heed early warning symptoms.

- 2. Avoid direct personal contact from the moment you recognize any of the symptoms of stage 1 until the sores disappear.

**DO NOT:**

- Have sex once you recognize an of the early symptoms.
- Scratch the blisters when they itch.
- Continually check out the progress of your sores by touching them.
- Touch your genital sores, even while urinating.
- Touch your lip sore, even while smoking a cigarette.
- Rest your chin in your hands while writing or thinking.
- Share anything that touches your mouth during an outbreak with anyone else (i.e. cigarette, toothbrush, drinking glass, eating utensils, etc.).

**NOTE:** Using sunscreen on the lips can help to prevent the formation of a herpes blister. Use SPF Factor 15 for maximum protection and apply before going out in the sun.

# WHAT FACTORS CONTRIBUTE TO THE DEVELOPMENT OF HERPES?

### THE ROLE OF THE IMMUNE SYSTEM

The key to the prevention and treatment of diseases is to maintain a healthy, well-functioning immune system. Unfortunately, due to a variety of causes, the human body can become nutrient deficient. Frequently, when essential nutrients are absent from the diet or poorly assimilated, immunity can become compromised. Impaired immunity can manifest itself as fatigue, irritability, and general susceptibility to disease and infections. In most cases, an outbreak of herpes can be preceded by a period of physical or emotional stress or in a body that has become disease debilitated. Like Candida, the herpes virus is considered an "opportunist" microbe and will invade human tissue whenever it become susceptible.

There are several ways to boost the immune system. They include:

1. *Eating properly*. Purdue University Nutrition Professor, Thomas Petro, Ph.D. states that, "it's not that certain nutrients affect the immune system, it's that every nutrient affects the immune system. Indeed, studies strongly suggest that each of the major vitamins (A,B,C,D and E) plays a significant role in protecting the human body against unfriendly organisms. Good food is vital for strong, resilient immunity. Eating a well-balanced diet which emphasizes of fresh fruits and vegetables, lean meat, beans and whole grain products, and lowfat dairy products helps to ensure that a wide variety of vitamins and minerals are available to the cells.

2. Exercise. Exercise can stimulate increased immunity to disease. In one experiment, rats were found to be more disease resistant after being injected with blood samples of people who had just exercised. Their body temperature increased slightly, the white blood cells multiplied, and other changes were noted, showing evidence that their immune systems were ready to battle any unwelcome microbe.

3. Other tips for strengthening immunity are: avoiding stressful situations, cultivating friendships, not smoking or drinking, and washing your hands often, as they are prime carriers of germs and viruses.

The human body has specific areas which are associated with the immune system. They involve: the nervous system, the blood, circulation, the bowels, and the thymus eland.

Strong nerves depend upon healthy blood and on nutritious food. We need to be aware of our nervous system and not wait until we have problems before we feed it properly.

When toxins are circulating around in the bloodstream they poison the cells, diminish immunity to disease, and cause a person to feel sick and rundown. It is extremely important, therefore, to keep our bloodstreams clean with proper food and herbs.

The circulatory system is responsible for increasing blood

supply to the heart muscles and the entire body. Good circulation is essential to the health of the immune system. However, when a person is under severe stress this circulatory network, and consequently, the immunity, will suffer. Reducing the intake of sugars and other refined carbohydrates, red meat, and white flour products, combined with increased activity (such as walking and jumping on a mini-trampoline) will help promote strong, high-caliber circulation.

Autointoxication or intestinal toxemia is a condition triggered by eating the wrong types and amounts of food which certain bacteria in the bowels will thrive upon. These bacteria then produce toxins which permeate the bloodstream, and then are carried via the blood to all parts of the body. Symptoms of auto-intoxication inlclude fatigue, nervousness gastrointestinal conditions, skin diseases, headaches, endocrine and circulatory disturbances, etc. Constipation causes the immune system to be poisoned. Correct diet, in which refined foods are avoided, will play a crucial role in alleviating this condition.

One of the most important components of the immune system is the tiniest. Located in your lower neck is the thymus gland, the master gland of the immune system. It is responsible for manufacturing T cells, white blood cells, commonly known as "T-lymphocytes". T-cells multiply in order to outnumber the enemy virus. They then migrate throughout the body, keeping a sharp 'watch' for virus infested cells. They then send a toxin which irritates the offended tissue and draws the macrophages or scavenger cells to join the war. Antibodies which are produced by organs having a large number of T cells adhere to the virus until the macrophages can devour them.

The thymus manufactures vital hormones involved in the immune process, one of them being "thymosin". The thymus gland will actually shrivel under stress, and nutrients, especially vitamin A and zinc, are needed to keep it functioning properly. Vitamin A increases the bodys ability to produce "antigens". (An antigen is an enemy substance to which the body reacts by producing antibodies.) Zinc deficiency has been linked to lack of immunity by lowering the activity of the T-cells. This, in turn, encourages the growth of infections, neoplastic and autoimmune diseases.

The mode of travel for lymphocytes throughout the body is

lymphatic fluid. Exercise promotes expansion and compression of lymph vessels, thus encouraging the lymphocytes and increasing immune function.

Nutrients play an integral role in building the immune system. Herbs, as well as the vitamins and minerals contained in them, are vital to our health. They supply the unique elements which the cells use to strengthen resistance to disease.

## THINGS TO AVOID

When you are afflicted with herpes, there are specific things to avoid. They include:
ACID PRODUCING FOODS: Tea, coffee, tobacco, alcohol, black pepper, mustard, hot spices, white vinegar, excess salt, aluminum baking powder, baking soda, jellies, sweet desserts, candy white bread, pastries, deep-fried foods, soft drinks, cola beverages, pizza, catsup, and mayonnaise.

TIGHT, CHAFING CLOTHING: This type of clothing in the genital area, does not allow the skin to breathe. Use cotton material.
ARGININE FOODS: Arginine is an amino acid. It is believed by many scientsts that arginine aggravates or promotes herpes outbreaks. Some foods which contain arginine are: Chocolate, cocoa, nuts, whole wheat, wheat gluten, barley, whole rye, buckwheat flour, (peanuts, pecans, almonds, cashews, walnuts), rice, corn, cottonseed whole oats.

STRESS: The body and mind react to stress by the tightening of muscles, impairment of blood flow to organs, constriction of the lungs, irregular heartbeat, high blood pressure, or altering of the immunity. Those people most susceptible to these symptoms are those who are always in a hurry, quick to anger, and always thinking of themselves. How we react to stress is a key element. Relax your mind by becoming involved in recreation, or unwind with a warm shower or soothing music. Other diversions are reading, watching TV, walking or jogging around the block. Aerobic and stretching exercises are excellent methods of alleviating stress. Other helps are: do not try to do too many things at a time, or too fast. Take relaxation breaks during a busy routine, and talk your problems out with someone close to you.

**DRUGS:** Avoid those drugs not recommended by your physician.

**HIGHLY REFINED CARBOHYDRATES:** These include white sugar, white flour, and most processed foods. The body requires large amounts of B vitamins in order to assimilate carbohydrates. Eating a lot of sugar diminishes the B vitamin supply in the body, eventually resulting in a deficiency. This can lead to chronic depression and mental disorders. Excessive sugar intake also contributes to both low blood sugar (hypoglycemia), and high blood sugar (diabetes), due to disturbances in the insulin metabolism.

## THINGS TO USE

**ALKALINE PRODUCING FOODS:** This includes whole grains, legumes, raw fruits (except citrus), vegetables, and herbs.

**LYSINE FOODS:** The amino acid lysine has been shown to alleviate the symptoms of herpes. These foods include chicken, fish and seafood, soy protein, soy beans, cottage cheese, baked beans, cow and goat milk products.

**POSITIVE ATTITUDE:** You may control your own mind and you have the power to feed it whatever thought impulses you choose. Many studies and much research has been conducted which proves that a positive state of mind boosts the body's immunity by releasing infection-fighting T-cells.

**VITAMIN E OIL:** When topically applied to herpes sores, this oil helps speed their healing.

**ESSENTIAL FATTY ACIDS:** Evening Primrose Oil, Black Currant Oil and Fish Lipids, provide these nutrients. It contains high amounts of PGE, a vitamin-like compound involved in proper function of the immune system. A shortage of PGE is believed to cause abnormal and harmful immune response. It stimulates the T-cells of the immune system to attack cancer. T-cells are the main mechanism of the immune system to protect the body from foreign cells, viruses, bacteria, fungi, and allergies.

**SULPHER BEARING AMINO ACIDS:** These amino acids are important constituents of the immune system framework. Through the sulphur they are able to make the mineral selenium available to the cells. We know that selenium is helpful in preventing cancer, and pulling heavy metals such as lead, mercury and cadmium from the body. They neutralize and eliminate potentially destructive free radicals which help in cell immunity.

The amino acids methionine, cysteine and taurine work as a team. During dieting methionine and cysteine will insure adequate taurine to protect the heart muscle from calcium and potassium loss.

**METHIONINE.** This amino acid helps keep hair, skin, nails, and joints healthy. It also helps cleanse the liver.

**CYSTEINE.** This amino acid helps protect the body from radiation, pollution, toxins, and toxic metals. Very effective when combined with Vitamin E.

**TAURINE.** This amino acid is critical to proper development in infants. Is very helpful when combined with zinc, especially for the eyes. It protects the loss of potassium in the heart muscle. Its synthesis is derived from two other amino acids, methionine and cysteine.

**ACIDOLPHILUS:** The acidophilus bacillus is a friendly organism which helps the body fight disease and restore health. Modern research has discovered that acidophilus kills the harmful bacteria strain of B. coli in the intestinal tract. Acidophilus breaks milk sugar down into lactic acid. Bacteria which produce putrefaction and gas cannot live in lactic acid. Acidophilus, taken internally, has been shown to be very beneficial in alleviating cold sores caused by herpes.

## HERBS FOR HERPES

**COMFREY:** Comfrey is one of the most valuable herbs known to botanical medicine. It has been used for centuries as a healer. It is rich in the amino acid, lysine, also B12, and vitamins A and C. It is high in calcium, potassium, phosphorus, and protein. It contains iron, magnesium, sulphur, copper, and zinc, as well as eighteen amino acids.

**ECHINACEA:** This herb stimulates immunity and increases the body's ability to fight infections. It contains vitamins A, E and C, iron, iodine, copper, sulphur, and potassium.

**FENNEL:** Fennel helps stabilize the nervous system and moves waste material out of the body. It has mucus countering and anticonvulsive properties. It contains potassium, sulphur and sodium.

**GARLIC:** Garlic has a rejuvenating effect on all body functions. It stimulates the lymphatic system to throw off toxins. It has been referred to as "nature's antibiotic" and Russian penicillin. This herb contains vitamins A and C. It also has selenium, which is closely related to vitamin E in biological activity. It contains sulphur, calcium, manganese, copper, and a lot of vitamin Bl. It has some iron and is high in potassium and zinc.

**GINGER:** This herb is very effective as a cleansing agent through the bowels and kidneys, and also through the skin. It contains protein, vitamins A, C, and B complex. It also contains, calcium, phosphorus, iron, sodium, potassium and magnesium.

**MULLEIN:** Mullein has the ability to loosen mucus and move it out of the body. It is high in iron, magnesium, potassium and sulphur. It contains vitamins A, D, and B complex.

**SWEET BIRCH (bark and leaves):** Birch contains natural properties for cleansing the blood. It is high in natural fluoride. It contains vitamins A, C, E, B1 and B2. It also has calcium, chlorine, copper, iron, magnesium, phosphorus, potassium, sodium and silicon.

**THYME:** Thyme destroys fungal infections, as in athlete's foot, and skin parasites such as crabs and lice. It has B complex, and vitamins C and D. It also contains a considerable amount of iodine, and some sodium, silicon and sulphur.

**WHITE WILLOW:** This herb has been called one of the essential first aid plants for the hiker. It has strong but benign antiseptic abilities for infected wounds, ulcerations, and eczema. We know of a case of a young woman who was often afflicted with cold sores in her mouth. A friend suggested she swish extract of white willow in her mouth. She did and it numbed the discomfort of the sores. Also, after doing this, the sores disappeared twice as fast as they normally did before.

# HERBS FOR THE NERVES

Research has produced evidence that the central nervous system is closely related to the immune system. The nervous system connects the body to the outside world and reacts to the environment. When one system fails to develop normally, the other is affected. Information is constantly being transmitted from the immune system to the brain and vice versa. The nervous system regulates the activities of all the other systems in the body and has three main divisions:

1. The central nervous system, which includes the brain and spinal cord.
2. The peripheral nervous system, made up of the nerves that extend out from the spinal cord and the base of the brain to the various of the body.
3. The autonomic nervous system, which regulates internal organs. These areas contain thousands of feet of nerves in the body. Strong nerves depend upon healthy blood and on the food consumed daily.

## NERVINE HERBS

**ALFALFA:** It is full of nutrients essential for the function of the central nervous system. Alfalfa contains the amino acid tryptophan, a nerve sedative.

**DANDELION:** This herb contains choline and linolenic acid. Choline is essential for the health of the myelin sheaths of the nerves.

**FENUGREEK:** This contains niacin, which helps strengthen the nerves and prevent migraine headaches.

**GOTU KOLA:** Gotu Kola is rich in B complex vitamins, which are essential to the maintenance of the nervous system. It feeds and nourishes the brain.

**HOPS:** Hops are rich in B vitamins to nourish the nerves. It is calming for the nerves, relaxes the body, and builds up the nervous system to protect the immune system from damage.

**KELP:** Kelp is rich in iodine and phosphorus, which are two of many wonderful minerals essential for nerve health. They are also excellent for the thyroid.

**LADY'S SLIPPER:** This herb acts as a tonic to the central nervous system. It is useful in all stressful situations. Good for emotional and anxiety states. Used to help with nervous pain.

**LOBELIA:** A wonderful herb with a combination of stimulation and re laxation properties. It has healing powers with the ability to remove congestion within the body.

**PARSLEY:** This herb contains polyunsaturated and saturated fatty acids, which have a positive influence on the nerves. It is also very high in vitamin A, which builds up the immune system.

**PASSION FLOWER:** It is a quieting, soothing herb for the central nervous system. It helps restore normal function. It has been used for insomnia, hysteria, and convulsions in children.

**SCULLCAP:** It will cleanse and rebuild malfunctional areas of the spinal cord. It is very useful in alleviating stress due to emotional conflicts, worry, disturbances of digestion, and circulation. Scullcap is an antispasmodic for tremors, spasms and restlessness. This herb is slow working but has no side effects and is safe and nourishing. It will aid in strengthening the spinal cord, is a liver cleanser, and helps prevent hardening of the arteries. It cleans the veins while it soothes the nerves.

**WOOD BETONY:** This herb acts as a stimulant fcr the nerves like black tea, but without any harmful effects. It strengthens the immune system and nervous system to protect against diseases.

**RED CLOVER:** It is useful as a tonic for the nerves and as a sedative for nervous exhaustion. It contains vitamins A, B-complex, C, F, P, and many minerals including magnesium, calcium, and copper.

## HERBS FOR CIRCULATION

The circulatory system is responsible for increasing blood supply to the heart muscles and the entire body. Good circulation is essential to the health of the immune system. However, when a person is under severe stress this circulatory network, and consequently the immunity, will suffer. With heart attacks and strokes claiming thousands of lives each year, we cannot ignore the importance of prevention. Proper diet, stress management, and exercise are three key elements involved in protecting the heart and ensuring that it does not stop before its time. Circulation is improved with the following herbs:

**CAPSICUM:** Capsicum is said to be unualled forwarding off diseases and equalizing blood circulation. It increases the heart action but not the blood pressure. It is said to prevent strokes and heart attacks. Capsicum is high in vitamins A and C, iron and calcium. It has vitamin G, magnesium, phosphorus, and sulphur. It has some B complex and is rich in potassium.

**GARLIC:** Garlic dissolves cholesterol in the bloodstream and stimulates the lymphatic system to throw off waste materials. It opens up the blood vessels and reduces blood pressure in hypertensive patients. This herb contains vitamins A and C, sulphur, calcium, manganese, copper, and is high in vitamin B 1, potassium, zinc and iron.

**GENTIAN ROOT:** Gentian is superior to other herbal aids because it does not cause constipation. It stimulates the circulation and strengthens the system, being one of the best stomach tonics in the herb kingdom. It is high in iron and contains B complex, especially inositol and niacin. It has vitamin F, manganese, silicon, sulphur, tin, lead, and zinc.

**HAWTHORN BERRIES:** Regular use of this herb strengthens the heart muscles. It has been used in preventing arteriosclerosis and in helping conditions like rapid and feeble heart action, heart valve defects, enlarged heart, angina pectoris and difficult breathing owing to ineffective heart action and lack of oxygen in the blood. Some herbalists recommend Hawthorn to use against diseases before actual symptoms are manifested. This herb is high in vitamins C and B complex. It contains sodium, silicon, phosphorus, and some iron, zinc, sulphur, nickel, tin, aluminum and beryllium.

**KELP:** Kelp is called a sustainer to the nervous system and the brain, helping it to function normally. It contains nearly 30 minerals. It is also rich in B complex vitamins. It contains vitamins A, C, E and G. It also contains anti-sterility vitamin S and has anti-hemmorhage vitamin K.

**LICORICE ROOT:** This herb has a stimulating action and counteracts stress. It contains vitamin E, phosphorus, B complex, biotin, niacin, and pantothenic acid. It also contains lecithin, manganese, iodine, chromium, and zinc.

**LECITHIN:** This nutrient dissolves cholesterol in the bloodstream.

## GLANDULAR HERBS

The glands regulate many major body functions. These functions interrelate with those in circulatory and nervous systems. Several glandular herbs are:

**GOLDEN SEAL:** Golden Seal has been recommended as a way of boosting a sluggish glandular system and promoting youthful hormone harmony. The action of the herb goes directly into the bloodstream and helps regulate the liver functions. It has a natural antibiotic ability to stop infection and kill poisons in the body. If a person has low blood sugar, substitute myrrh instead of golden seal. This herb contains vitamins A and C. It also contains vitamin B complex, E, F, calcium, copper, potassium, phosphorus, manganese, iron, zinc, and sodium.

**SIBERIAN GINSENG:** This herb acts as an overall tonic which stimulates mental and physical health. It strengthens the adrenal glands. It increases energy, improves vision, and helps the nervous and cardiovascular systems. It is very beneficial for increasing body resistance to stress and infections. Ginseng contains vitamins A and E. It also contains thiamine, riboflavin, B12, niacin, calcium, iron, phosphorus, sodium, silicon, potassium, manganese and sulphur.

**BURDOCK:** It aids the pituitary gland in releasing an ample supply of protein to help adjust hormone balance in the body. This herb contains vitamin C, iron, vitamin A, P, Bcomplex, vitainin E, PABA, and small amounts of sulphur, silicon, copper, iodine and zinc.

**ECHINACEA:** This herb helps to restore the glands to proper functioning. It is considered a nontoxic way of cleansing the system. Echinacea contains vitamins A, E, and C, iron, iodine, copper, sulphur, and potassium.

**SARSAPARILLA:** Sarsaparilla is a valuable herb used in glandular balance formulas. Its stimulating properties are noted for increasing the metabolic rate. It contains B complex, vitamins A, C and D. It also contains iron, manganese, sodium, silicon, sulphur, copper, zinc, and iodine.

**BLACK WALNUT:** Helps restore the thyroid, liver, lymphatics, skin, muscles, reproductive and intestinal areas. It is excellent to help bal ance the functioning of these areas. It is rich in vitamin B15 and man ganese. Black walnut contains magnesium, silica, protein, calcium, phosphorvs, iron and potassium.

**CHAPARRAL:** It is a potent healer, and tones up the system and rebuilds tissues. It is a strong antioxidant, antitumor agent, painkiller, and antiseptic. It is one of the best herbal antibiotics. It is high in protein, potassium, and sodium. It also contains silicon, tin, alumi num, sulphur, chlorine, and barium.

**RED CLOVER BLOSSOMS:** This herb helps improve liver function and eliminate poisons. It is good for coughs, weak chest, wheezing, bronchitis, and lack of vitality. It contains selenium, cobalt, nickel, manganese, sodium, and tin. It is rich in magnesium, calcium, and copper.

## HERBS FOR THE SKIN

**ALOE VERA:** This herb cleans, soothes and heals. It contains calcium, potassium, sodium, manganese, magnesium, iron, lecithin, and zinc.

**COMEREY:** Comfrey helps in the calcium/phosphorus balance by promoting strong bones and healthy skin. It is rich in vitamins A and C, calcium, potassium, phosphorus, and protein. It contains iron, magnesium, sulphur, copper and zinc, as well as eighteen amino acids. It is a good source of the amino acid, lysine, usually lacking in diets which contain no animal products.

**GOLDEN SEAL:** Golden Seal is valuable for all mucous conditions, in the nasal area, bronchial tubes, throat, intestines, stomach or bladder. It has the ability to heal mucus membranes anywhere in the body. It contains vitamins A, C,

B complex, E, F, calcium, copper, potassium, phosphorus, manganese, iron, zinc and sodium.

**MYRRH:** It is a powerful antiseptic on the mucus membranes. It helps soothe inflammation and speeds the healing process. The essential oils contain antiseptic properties and when used as a tincture mixed with water, it is excellent as a gargle for sore throat. It helps in waste elimination.

**BAYBERRY:** It is used as a tonic, stimulating the system to help raise vitality and resistance to disease, and at the same time to aid digestion, nutrition, and build the blood.

**OAT (straw):** Oatstraw is a powerful stimulant and is rich in body building materials. It is an important skin and membrane aid, because it is rich in organic silicon. It is also high in calcium, and contains phosphorus and vitamins A, B1, B2 and E.

## MINERALS FOR THE IMMUNE SYSTEM

**CALCIUM:** This element is healing to the body. It prevents heavy metals from accumulating in the body. Without adequate calcium, the body absorbs heavy metals. Calcium is destroyed by aspirin, coffee, stress, lack of exercise, lack of magnesium, lack of hydrochloric acid, mineral oil and oxalic acid.

**CHROMIUM:** Although only needed in small amounts by the body, this mineral is critical in fighting infections.

**IODINE:** This helps the thyroid gland produce the hormone thyroxine. It also helps the body absorb vitamin A. Lack of this nutrient can cause loss of interest in living and can promote a tendency to get fat.

**MAGNESIUM:** When a person is deficient in this mineral they can experience a personality change. Magnesium produces properdin, a blood protein that fights invading viruses and bacteria. It is destroyed by alcohol, diuretics, white sugar, white flour, and a high protein diet.

**MANGANESE:** It activates enzymes that work with vitamin C. As a team, they fight toxins and free radicals. It also stimulates the release of histamine, which protects the immune system. It is destroyed by high meat intake, excess phosphorus, and calcium.

**SELENIUM:** This mineral is critical and is needed in only small amounts in the body, therefore, is considered to be a trace nutrient. 300 mcg. daily are considered safe for human consumption. Cancer rates are lowest in regions with selenium-rich soil. Selenium inhibits breast, skin, liver, and colon cancer. Selenium and vitamin E work together to protect the body's cells. It is essential to the body's production of glutathione peroxidase, an enzyme that disarms free radicals.

## VITAMINS FOR THE IMMUNE SYSTEM

The following three vitamins are important for many reasons. However, they are most renowned for their antioxidant qualities. An antioxidant helps to protect cells from being robbed of oxygen, which is essential to their functioning. Without adequate oxygen, cells can deteriorate and die. Or it can impair them and make them sick enough to reproduce erratically. This can lead to disorders like cancer. Free radicals smother cells so that oxygen cannot be properly utilized.

**VITAMIN A:** Vitamin A increases resistance to infections. Deficiencies increase chances of viral, bacterial and protozoal invasions, and their severity. It is an essential nutrient to protect against cancer. Laboratory evidence shows that vitamin A is able to suppress chemically induced tumors. This vitamin is involved in the maintenance of epithelial linings and mucous membranes, which are the first places that are penetrated by foreign organisms. Vitamin A protects against the effects of all types of pollution. The protection of vitamin A seems to be most evident among smokers. It reduces susceptibility to respiratory problems, i.e., colds, sinusitis, asthma, bronchitis, ear infections, and cystic fibrosis. It increases immunity against environmental pollution such as pesticides and herbicides. It works with zinc for optimum efficiency. Vitamin A is destroyed by high heat.

**VITAMIN E:** This vitamin prevents the oxidized state that cancer cells thrive in. It deactivates the free radicals that promote cellular damage leading to malignancy. Deficiencies of vitamin

E depress general resistance to disease. Processing and storage destroys some of the vitamin E content of most foods.

**VITAMIN C:** This vitamin plays a role in the formation of connective tissue in the body. It also helps the body's absorption of iron. More importantly, however, vitamin C has shown even more poweiful effects through animal, human and test-tube studies. They've demonstrated that this vitamin can activate white blood cells to battle foreign substances and increase the production of interferon, the body's antivirus protein. Vitamin C also has the ability to kill disease inducing bacteria. Vitamin C can be affected by exposure to light, long-term storage of foods, heat and canning.

## B VITAMINS

B vitamins protect the immune and nervous systems. They help build blood, protect the body against infection and help produce antibodies. They increase production of hydrochloric acid for digestion, and are very vital in helping stabilize mood swings. These are the vitamins that support the immune system by reducing the impact of stress in one's life.

**B1 (Thiamine):** This B complex vitamin is helpful for cell respiration, metabolism of carbohydrates, a healthy heart and proper growth of the body.

**B2 (Riboflavin):** It is used by the body to metabolize proteins and lipids; supplies oxygen to the cells, and is used by the skin and nails. It is especially needed during stressful situations.

**B3 (Niacin):** This nutrient stimulates circulation. It aids memory function, releases histamines and helps in hyperactivity. It is an excellent vitamin for the nerves. It is essential for brain metabolism. It reduces tension, fatigue, depression and insomnia.

**B5 (Pantothenic Acid):** It protects against respiratory infections and is a natural tranquilizer.

**B6 (Pyridoxine):** The body uses B6 in hormone and antibody production, in the synthesis of DNA and RNA and in the metabolism of fat, protein and carbohydrates. It is nature's diuretic and is very useful in menstruation and the water

gained at this time. It is excellent for insomnia.
**B12:** This nutrient increases the body's resistance to infection. A person especially needs this vitamin when fatigued. It helps form red blood cells, and helps prevent constipation.
**B15:** It is used for the proper functioning skin, nerves, bone marrow, and reproductive glands. It helps metabolize carbohydrates and protein.
**CHOLINE:** This helps keep the nerve coverings (myelin) healthy; aids in production of acetycholine (a neurotransmitter), and helps the body utilize fat and cholesterol.
**FOLIC ACID:** It is used for red blood cell formation and the synthesis of DNA and RNA.
**INOSITOL:** Works with choline and is vital for nourishment of the brain. It has been shown to help reduce fat in the liver.
**PABA (Paraaminobenzoic Acid):** This vitamin protects the body against free radicals and is part of the folic acid molecule.

## OTHER HELPS:

**PAU D'ARCO (Taheebo) TEA:** This herb, which is a powerful immune builder, is excellent as a tea.
**COMEREY TEA:** This contains the amino acid lysine, which helps prevent eruption of 'cold sores'.

## CASE HISTORY

Jo Ann is a vivacious single mother of five children. She has had many trials and hardships in her life, but always seems to bounce back.

Her problems began several years ago when she was eighteen years old. She came down with mononucleosis and hepatitis, both at the same time. She almost died because the combination of diseases infected all of her organs and caused her spleen to enlarge. She later learned that this was due to the EpsteinBarr virus.

Years later, soon after she was divorced from an alcoholic husband, stress caused the Epstein Barr to surface again. She was trying to support her family, but was constantly missing work, due to sickness.

At one point, she was flat in bed for six weeks straight. She was so weak she had to have her oldest daughter help her walk across the hall about six steps to go to the bathroom. There were six stairs from her bedroom to the living room and she couldn't even go from one to the other. She was totally exhausted and walking was a formidable task.

One doctor told her that she had multiple sclerosis and became very upset with her when she expressed a desire to get well. "You'd better face the fact that you may not be able to ever work again!" he almost yelled.

There were days she slept twelve to sixteen hours at a stretch, she was so exhausted.

The doctor who told her she had multiple sclerosis put her on 'antidepressants'. He said, "I don't know exactly why these work but my multiple sclerosis patients seem to do better when they are taking them." Jo Ann felt even more tired and weak after taking them and told the doctor they weren't doing her any good.

A friend of Jo Ann's asked her if she would like to try herbs. Jo Ann didn't know anything about herbs but agreed to try them. "What could it hurt?" she asked. "I've tried everything else." Her friend put her on a regime of fresh fruits and vegetables (mostly vegetables), and told her to quit drinking cokes. She had her drink grape juice daily with liquid chlorophyll and a red clover combination extract. Jo Ann took an herbal liver formula, B complex, Pau D'Arco, an herbal blood cleansing formula and an herbal laxative with Cascara Sagrada. She also took vitamin E, cod liver oil and evening primrose oil. Where before she thought she was dying, within twenty four hours of taking the herbs and vitamins she felt her mind clearing and she was more alert. By the third day she had more strength and by the fourth day she was going down the stairs and going out grocery shopping.

Where the doctors said they couldn't do anything for her, she has been helped with the nutritional approach. She found out she had Candida albicans and is taking steps to eradicate that also. One nutritionally oriented doctor told a friend of hers who also has the EpsteinBarr virus that he believes Epstein Barr is Candida albicans "gone haywire". Jo Ann still has a ways to go before she is 100% well, but compared to what happened before, she is already 100% better, thanks to the herbal nutritional route.

## TRUE TALES

One man took extract of Lady's Slipper, B complex and apple cider vinegar for his case of herpes induced shingles. The shingles went away within a couple of weeks, much to the astonishment of the doctors.

Two ladies were at a convention. A person they knew gave them each a "hello" kiss, and two days later they came down with the beginnings of cold sores. They each applied ice to the area for 30 minutes, took vitamin A and chewable vitamin C. They opened a vitamin C capsule, dissolved vitamin E into it, and applied it to the affected area. The fever blister went away and never developed!

# MENUS AND RECIPES

Many of the following recipes are taken from *Today's Healthy Eating* by Louise Tenney. The recipes marked with an * are included in this booklet.

## SEVEN DAY SAMPLE MENU

#1 Breakfast
    Yogurt and Fruit*

#1 Lunch
    Spinach and Mushroom Salad*
    Steamed carrot slices with butter

#1 Supper
    Baked Rice and Millet*
    Steamed green beans
    1 cup Comfrey Tea

#2 Breakfast
    Poached egg
    Sliced peach

#2 Lunch
    Broccoli Quiche*
    1 cup Comfrey Tea

#2 Supoer
    Baked fish (of choice), in butter
    Sprout and Seed Salad*
    1 cup fresh carrot juice

#3 Breakfast
    Steamed yam (excellent cold with honey and cinnamon)

#3 Lunch
    Brussels Sprouts Casserole*
    1 cup fresh vegetable juice (of choice)

#3 Supper
    Layered Vegetable Salad*
    Steamed chicken breast, cut in chunks

| | |
|---|---|
| #4 Breakfast | Omelette with mushrooms, bell pepper, onions, and crab cheese.<br>1 cup Comfrey Tea |
| #4 Lunch | Tuna sandwich<br>Carrot sticks |
| #4 Supper | Dried Pea Soup*<br>Baked potato, with sour cream and chives |
| #5 Breakfast | Super Breakfast Cereal*<br>1 cup Comfrey Tea |
| #5 Lunch | Green Salad*<br>1 boiled egg |
| #5 Supper | Stuffed Peppers*<br>1 cup fresh carrot juice |
| #6 Breakfast | 1 cantaloupe cut into chunks, mix with seedless green grapes, strawberries |
| #6 Lunch | Chop Suey and Vegetables*<br>Steamed chicken breast, cut into chunks |
| #6 Supper | Steamed broccoli |

# RECIPES

## FRUIT AND YOGURT

2 C. yogurt
2 C. fresh or frozen blue berries or strawberries
2 ripe bananas
1 apple, grated
pure maple syrup
unsweetened coconut, shredded

Fold fruit into yogurt, sweeten with maple syrup to taste. Garnish with coconut.

## SPINACH AND MUSHROOM SALAD

1 bunch spinach
1 1/2 C. sliced raw mushrooms
1 T. parmesan cheese, grated
1 1/2 tsp. garlic
1 1/2 C. croutons

Wash spinach thoroughly, dry and tear into small pieces. Add all ingredients and toss with a French dressing.

## BAKED RICE AND MILLET

1 1/2 C. cooked brown rice
1 1/2 C. cooked millet
2 eggs, beaten
2 C. milk
2 T. butter
2 T. tamari soy sauce
1 C. chopped nuts
1 C. chopped sunflower seeds

Mix all ingredients. Pour into 1 1/2 quart casserole dish. Bake 10 minutes at 350° F.

## BROCCOLI QUICHE

2 C. broccoli  
1 C. fresh sliced mushrooms  
1 1 2 6. onions, chopped  
1 clove garlic, pressed  
2 T. butter  
6 eggs, beaten  

1 C. half & half  
2 1/2 T. Swiss cheese, grated  
1 1/2 tsp. mineral salt  
1 1/2 tsp. nutmeg  
1 tsp. basil  

Saute' broccoli, onions, and mushrooms in butter. Cook until onions are transparent. Mix eggs, cream, cheese, salt, nutmeg, basil, parsley and vegetable seasoning. Mix all ingredients in a buttered twoquart casserole. Bake for 30 minutes at 3500F.

## BRUSSELS SPROUTS CASSEROLE

1 C. Brussels sprouts, steamed  
1 C. red cabbage, chopped  
2 red onions, chopped  
1 C. carrots, sliced and steamed  

1 C. potatoes, skins on, diced and steamed  
2 T. mineral bouillon  
1 T. mineral salt  
1 tsp. kelp  
2 T. olive oil  
1 C. tomato juice  

Combine steamed Brussels sprouts, carrots and potatoes. Add all other ingredients and cover with tomato juice. Cook in oven for 30 minutes at 350° F.

## MILLET CASSEROLE

Put two cups of cooked millet in a buttered baking dish. Add 6 chopped green onions, 1 1 2 cup grated carrots, one small green pepper, 2 medium chopped tomatoes and 1 cup chopped mushrooms. Add vegetable seasoning or herbs. Mix all together and top with 1 cup grated cheese. Bake in oven just until it is warm all the way through.

## LAYERED VEGETABLE SALAD

(This is a complete salad meal. It contains easily digestible quality protein, along with vitamins, minerals and live enzymes.

4 C. romaine and leaf lettuce
112 C. ground sunflower seeds
1 small green pepper, diced
1 C. alfalfa sprouts

1 avocado, sliced
1 large tomato, diced
1 C. buckwheat sprouts
1 small cucumber, diced

Break up the lettuce and use half of it on the bottom of a salad bowl. Layer half of the other ingredients, add the rest of the lettuce and then another layer of the same ingredients.

## DRIED PEA SOUP

1 C. dried split peas
4 C. pure water, cold
1 medium onion, minced
1 C. celery, chopped;
2 small carrots, grated

2 T. chopped parsley
11/2 C. nut cream
1 tsp. vegetable salt
or kelp

Cook the peas in water after soaking overnight. Cook with vegetables for about two hours. When done, add nut cream and seasoning.

## SUPER BREAKFAST CEREAL

11/2 C. oatmeal
1 C. plain yogurt
2 T. orange juice
1 T. honey
11/2 C. raisins

1 T. sesame seeds
11/2 C. chopped
11/2 C. chopped apples
11/2 C. sliced bananas

Fold all ingredients together. Sunflower seeds can be substituted for sesame seeds, or pecans for almonds.

## GREEN SALAD

1 C. spinach
1 C. red lettuce
1 C. romaine lettuce
1 C. watercress

1 C. celery, sliced
1 1/4 C. green onions, chopped
3 T. parsley, chopped

Serve with your favorite dressing.

## STUFFED PEPPERS

6 green peppers, large
2 7. butter
4 small onions
1 C. cooked brown rice
1 C. cooked millet

1 C. almonds, ground
1 C. cheese, grated
4 eggs, beaten
Vegetable seasoning to taste

Remove the pulp and seeds of the peppers. Saute' onion in butter. Mix all the other ingredients with the onions and butter. Stuff each pepper until full. Arrange the peppers open end up in a baking dish. Pour water into the dish to barely cover the bottom. Bake for 30 minutes at 350°F. Leftover stuffing can be used for a casserole.

## CHOP SUEY VEGETABLES

1 C. green and red peppers sliced diagonally
1 C. celery, sliced
112 &. onions, sliced
1 small can water water chestnuts
1 &. bamboo shoots
1 7. sesame seeds

1 C. bean sprouts
1 C. mushrooms, sliced
1 1/8 tsp. ginger
2 cloves garlic, minced
4 T. butter
4 tsp. tamari (soy sauce)

Cook vegetables lightly and serve over cooked brown rice or millet Vegetables should be crunchy.

## SWEET POTATO CASSEROLE

2 T. mashed, cooked, sweet potatoes
1 T. mashed bananas
1 1/3 T. yogurt or sour cream
1 egg
1 1/2 tsp. mineral salt
2 T. pure maple syrup

Blend all ingredients together. Beat until smooth. Bake in a buttered casserole dish at 350°F for 20 minutes. Serves 4-6.

## BANANA SHAKE

1 large banana
1 T. fruit and berry juice or apple juice
1 T. protein powder
4 ice cubes
2 heaping T. plain yogurt gun
1 T. whey powder
fresh strawberries

Combine banana, juice, protein powder, yogurt, whey powder, and strawberries and mix in blender. Add ice cubes to make it thick like a milk shake.

## POTATO SOUP

4 large potatoes
3 C. water
2 7. raw cashew butter
1 small onion
4 stalks celery, chopped
1 1/2 &. fresh chopped parsley
1 tsp. vegetable salt

Steam potatoes with skins on in the water. Remove skin from potatoes and mash through dicer. Dissolve nut butter in 1 cup of warm pure water. Put all other ingredients together and cook in double boiler for about 20 minutes.